AF492299

AMAZING NUTRITIONAL AND VEGGIE POWER

Appolinaire LIMA

CONTENTS

DISCLAIMER

This book was created only for educational purposes. Every attempt has been taken to make this book as thorough and accurate as possible.

However, typographical or content errors may occur. Furthermore, the information in this book is only current as of the date of publication. Therefore, this booklet should be used as a guide — not as the definitive source.

The goal of this booklet is to teach. The author and publisher make no warranty that the content in this e-book is comprehensive and are not liable for any mistakes or omissions.

The author and publisher will have no duty or obligation to any person or entity for any loss or damage caused or alleged to be caused by this book, whether directly or indirectly.

CHAPTER ONE :
WHY ARE VITAMINS
AND MINERALS
THE ANSWER?

Many of us wish we had more energy, stronger abs, and greater attention. Similarly, we frequently wish we had better skin or hair. We hope we could sleep better at night and wish it were a little simpler to wake up (by the way, those last two statements are connected!).

This has brought about the emergence of numerous industries, all constructed around assisting us to feel, look, and perform higher. We spend large amounts of coins on skin care merchandise, on sleep dietary supplements, and on gym memberships. We attempt all types of loopy matters, whether that's lying on a bed of mild spikes to enhance sleep (yes, that's an actual thing!), carrying blue-blocking shades all day, or sporting electricity recuperation crystals (that are approximately as powerful as wishing in reality tough!).

We try this stuff due to the fact we're seeking out solutions, and we're determined. We're inclined to try anything. And we hope, each time, that we're about to come across the solution and liberate our complete capacity.

We hope that one among these items will offer the solution and help us feel remarkable as we recognize that we absolutely can do it. however very few of those techniques make any substantial difference.

The trouble? We're overcomplicating subjects. And this is basically because of the huge quantity of advertising that gets thrown at us on an everyday basis. In reality, enhancing the way you look and experience is quite simple: it's about the fundamentals!

Don't forget what may be very likely to be your modern lifestyle and your current weight-reduction plan. Improve your hand if any of those points apply to you :
• You don't manage your five end result and greens an afternoon
• You consume a variety of processed ingredients and ready food
• You go to the fitness center 3 times a week or much less — and aren't mainly mobile the rest of the time
• You don't get sufficient sleep
• you are in a country of persistent stress due to paintings, circle of relatives, and monetary pressures
• You spend a lot of your loose time on the sofa, watching cartoons
• You spend greater than 8 hours a day searching at a laptop display, with a hunched back, gazing a vibrant display screen
• You spend slightly any time outdoors
• You drink contaminated faucet water
• You breathe harmful smog-crammed air.

This is a substitute for a bleak image, however it's true for a lot of us. We don't eat sufficient veggies, we don't sleep, we gorge on sugary meals, and we're harassed all the time. Then we wonder why we don't experience a hundred %!

Although you acquire most of these items right, the fact is that our current existence is simply surely terrible for our fitness.

This is true right all the way down to the truth that most people are too comfy — we have become "tailored" to a comfortable, domesticated way of life, and consequently our bodies have forgotten how to address stress or issues.

Take going outdoors as an instance. Most folks simply don't do that enough, this means that we aren't getting the essential stimulus of sunlight, which helps to inspire the frame to provide diet D, which in turn regulates things like hormone production, sleep, temper... even the urge for food!

Without that crucial input (called an "outside zeitgebers" inside the scientific literature) our frame loses some of its natural rhythm and positive strategies are interrupted.

However, then there's the large benefit of being bloodless. Even if the sun isn't out, being outside facilitates to boost testosterone levels, strengthen our immune system, or even enhance our potential to regulate our very own body temperature.

Is it any wonder we continually experience "stuffy" whilst we by no means educate this part of our fitness?

Even spending time barefooted in the world (which trains tiny muscular tissues inside the foot), even diving into water and maintaining our breath (which trains our lungs and improves our CO2 balance)... these are all matters our bodies crave. And we aren't giving them that.
And our bodies are deteriorating massively as a result. Examine a wolf within the wild to an obese, spoiled home dog. Is that more healthy?

You are that home canine. Plus an extremely worrying way of life and absence of sleep...

BEGINNING WITH VEGGIES AND FRUITS IS THE ANSWER.

Beginning with fruits and vegetables is the answer. Why?

Well, it's all superb and nicely I am telling you which you have to be running out at some stage in the day, and which you must be consuming perfectly, and that you ought to be taking long swims in freezing bloodless water inside in the morning. Hassle is, we don't have time for that and our bodies are actually so maladaptive that they wouldn't handle it.

Even fixing your weight loss program – eliminating all that unwanted processed food, lowering the wide variety of overall energy, getting extra fiber, reducing simple carbs... it's a number of paintings and might get pretty complicated. That's why the first-rate location to start is by way of solving one of the most important troubles with present day lifestyles. This is: the dearth of micronutrients.

Micronutrients are nutrients, minerals, amino acids, fatty acids, antioxidants, and other lively substances in our meals that our body makes use of for an extensive variety of various purposes.

What many humans don't recognize is that we literally are what we devour. You listen to this plenty, but many human beings expect that it is a sort of metaphor. However, no: your frame takes within the nutrients which you consume after which it uses those nutrients to absolutely rebuild your frame.

For instance, your bones are made partly from calcium, and magnesium. These also help to bolster your connective tissue (tendons and ligaments), your tooth, and your nails. Connective tissues in addition benefit from the likes of collagen (observed in bone broth) which additionally allows to improve your pores and skin.

If most effective you may get greater fruit and greens to your weight loss program then, you will end up the healthiest and handiest model of yourself. And that during turn may then give you the electricity and strength of will to do the relaxation.

Fruits and veggies can even supercharge your metabolism, supporting you to burn through plenty greater fat!

As we can see within the relaxation of this book, fixing your consumption of end result and greens doesn't want to be tough. In case you are strategic, then making just a few easy adjustments can remodel your health and well-being.
This book may even define a few of the other extraordinary and complicated ways wherein culmination can enhance your fitness and performance — some of that are surely transformative to the manner you appear and feel.

You'll know exactly which end result and greens you need to remedy any of your current maladies, and you'll realize precisely the way to get them.
Let us get to it.

CHAPTER 2: AN INTRODUCTION TO NUTRIENTS

Earlier than we cross in addition, allows study more intently the particular benefits of culmination and veggies. And of course, the first region to begin is by way of searching on the nutrition content material.

It is possible to wonder if you recognize that nutrients had been observed much less than 100 years ago. Until they had been officially determined, doctors knew that positive meals helped with certain physical conditions, however they did not now understand why.

As an example, the British army carried a supply of limes as early as 1975 due to the fact that medical doctors had determined that consuming a certain amount every day, or consuming the juice, stopped sailors from getting scurvy.

But, it became now not until 1912 that Casimir Funk, working in the UK then later within the united states got here up with the term "vitamins," which later became vitamins.

The examination of vitamins has improved considering that point, and while most of us know the names of the most common vitamins, we won't constantly understand what they do. There are styles of vitamins. Those are fat soluble nutrients and water-soluble nutrients.

Fat soluble nutrients are the ones that the body is capable of. Which means in case you do not use all the nutrients that you eat, they can be saved in the body for use while the frame is in need of them.

The plain gain of fats soluble vitamins is that if your weight loss program is quickly missing this type of vitamins, you're much less probable to go through a deficiency. The downside of these types of nutrients is that if you consume an excessive amount of or considered one of them, then your body is not able to flush out the excess and you could suffer from a diet overdose.

FATS SOLUBLE NUTRIENTS

The most typically recognized fat soluble vitamins are vitamin A, vitamin D, vitamin E and vitamin K.

Vitamin A allows to hold the pores and skin moisturized, as well as ensuring that the mucus membranes continue to be wet, supple and easy. It also allows healthy eyesight in low light, in addition to keeping the reproductive system healthy and selling wholesome bone boom.

Vitamin A encompasses complete milk, butter, eggs and liver. A form of vitamin A, carotenoids are observed in red, yellow and Turkish green vegetable and fruit.

Vitamin D is critical for the body to soak up calcium. Therefore, it is chargeable for healthy enamel and bones, just like calcium. But, both are needed and paintings together. Vitamin D is frequently brought to 'fortified' foods consisting of fats spreads and cereals. It's also referred to as the light diet as the primary supply of diet D comes from daylight.

Vitamin E is accountable for retaining healthful muscle tissues, anxious gadgets and reproductive machines. It's also an antioxidant. Being fat soluble, it is saved inside the body and might assist to defend frame cells from the outcomes of loose radicals, which might be unfavorable to different body cells.

Sources of vitamin E encompass complete grains, nuts, wheat-germ oil and inexperienced leafy vegetables. Overdosing on nutrients is thought to be risky. Diet ok is in particular liable for blood clotting. Without it, each time you cut yourself you'll be in chance of bleeding to dying.

This nutrition also makes kidney tissues and bones. Assets of diet k consist of liver, cheese, cereals, Turkish green leafy vegetables and fruit. It is also made inside the intestines by means of friendly bacteria.

Water-soluble vitamins can not be saved in the frame. Which means if you eat an excessive amount of this sort of nutrients, the amount that isn't always used is excreted through urine. The benefit of water-soluble nutrients is that you are unlikely to suffer from an overdose.

The drawback of these nutrients is that you may want to take in larger amounts as it can not be stored. If your food regimen is deficient in the sort of nutrients, even for a short time, you can go through signs and symptoms of vitamin deficiency as a result, there may be no back up supply stored for your body.

WATER SOLUBLE VITAMINS

The maximum usually recognized water-soluble vitamins are diet C, and the complete group of B nutrients. Vitamin C is also called ascorbic acid. It helps to preserve the body's connective tissues, that is, the muscle, fats, and bone framework.

It additionally helps to heal wounds via rushing up the production of recent cells, is an antioxidant, and enables the frame to absorb iron. Any other feature of nutrition C is to protect the body's immune system enabling it to fight infection.

Sources of vitamin C consist of fruit, fruit juices and veggies. The B organization of vitamins consists of B1 or thiamine, B2 or riboflavin, B3 or niacin, B6 or pyridoxine and B12 or cyanocobalamin. This institution of nutrients is largely concerned with retaining the body functioning nicely.

Vitamin B1 is essential in supporting the frame to metabolize energy from fats, alcohol and carbohydrates. Resources of this diet are lean red meat, unrefined cereals, seeds and nuts.

B2 enables the frame to use and digest carbohydrates and proteins and keeps a healthy appetite. Resources of B2 include fish, rooster, meat, milk and eggs. Brewers yeast is a good supply of this diet, as are Turkish leafy veggies.

B3 is vital for proper boom and permitting oxygen to go with the flow through body tissues. It is also liable for keeping a wholesome urge for food. Assets of nutrition B3 consist of fortified bread and cereals and meat.

B6 is liable for obtaining vitamins and electricity from the food we devour. It facilitates coronary heart disorder with the aid of disposing of extra homocysteine from the blood. Assets of B6 encompass soy beans, nuts, eggs, entire grains, fish, lamb, port, chicken and milk.

B12 enables the formation of healthy pink blood cells. It additionally enables the frame to transmit messages among the body's nerve cells, allowing us to hear, flow, assume and perform normal activities. It is made by organisms in the body's small intestine. This nutrition is delivered to many foods, inclusive of cereals, and even though it is a water-soluble nutrition, it may be stored within the liver. Sources of B12 include hen, fish, milk, meat and eggs.

The best manner of making sure that you absorb enough water-soluble and fats soluble nutrients is to devour a balanced weight loss program. If you assume that you will be poor in some vitamins, you have to consult a medical doctor for advice.

CHAPTER 3: AN ADVENT TO MINERALS AND DIFFERENT EXCEPTIONAL NUTRIENTS IN FRUITS AND VEGGIES

While fruits are generally filled with vitamins, minerals generally tend to come more from our vegetables — although make no mistake, each fruit and vegetable are packed with both.

So, a very good query to start with is probably: what's the difference between a vitamin and a mineral ?

While nutrients are organic and thereby are typically quite risky (they can be broken down by the likes of warmth, air, and acid), minerals are conversely inorganic. In reality, a mineral can certainly be a metal or a rock — something you will never actually think of as being an essential building block in what makes you. However, minerals are crucial to the wholesome function of the human body. Iron for example is an important mineral that the body uses to make hemoglobin — the crimson blood cells that tour across the body carrying oxygen.

Without this method, it might be impossible to provide electricity around the frame for the limitless critical functions that cross on — together with respiratory, digesting, and more.

Usually, minerals tend to have a barely extra essential position within the structural factors of the human frame — and the more difficult elements. For example, minerals shape bones, tendons, and ligaments.

Minerals also play a function in conduction, but. The body is powered by means of power in spite of everything, and maintaining the best price is crucial for the wholesome characteristic of our muscular tissues and mind.

That's why an incorrect balance of sodium and potassium can cause cramping, because the frame is unable to send messages successfully to the muscular tissues. Likewise, a lack of calcium can lessen power as it is needed to handle the price within the muscle cells.

Did you recognize it? You could inform the distinction between a fruit and vegetable based totally at the seed/stone. Vegetables don't have them! Ingredients which have unexpected categorizations encompass: tomatoes (fruit), coconut (fruit), avocado (fruit), and cucumber (fruit).

OTHER ESSENTIAL MICRONUTRIENTS

As well as being rich in vitamins and minerals, fruits and vegetables are also a wealthy source of the two other essential vitamins. The opposite important vitamins are: critical fatty acids, and critical amino acids.

The term "critical" means that these materials can't be synthesized within the frame, and so consequently must be obtained from our diet. And possibly this has to also be a clue as to how large a trouble it is that 99% of us are not getting them that manner!
So, what do those vitamins do?

Well, amino acids are basically the building blocks of proteins. We get a variety of these from meat, and our bodies will then ruin down those constituent parts on the way to rebuild our tissue. As we saw at the start of this e-book, we literally are what we eat!

This is why amino acids and proteins by extension are so important for bodybuilders and athletes seeking to construct muscle.

Research indicates that the best balance for athletes is 1 gram of protein for each 1lb of body weight. Protein additionally has other advantages — it's far more difficult to transform into fats for instance, and it has a thermionic effect that means that virtually digesting it'll genuinely burn calories!

As a result, many humans will be tough at work searching for assets of protein from meat and could eat big quantities of chicken to construct larger muscle tissues. This will grow to be difficult work! However, what they overlook is that vegetables or even culmination additionally contain protein (although veggies are barely superior in this sense).

Don't simply matter the protein you obtain from that protein shake and shook, reflect on consideration on how a great deal is in the broccoli at the side of the fowl.

Amino acids additionally play a host of other roles within the frame and are used to provide digestive enzymes, neurotransmitters (brain chemicals) and plenty greater. They also can do things together while developing.

Ultimately, culmination and vegetables include essential fatty acids. Those are important fats that help us to soak up other fruits and veggies, and additionally serve quite a number of extra beneficial blessings — which includes improving mind function (the brain is made from a huge quantity of fats!).

Omega 3 is one of the most powerful crucial fatty acids there may be and has a large host of fantastic benefits. Regularly, we think about omega three as being something we get from fish, but in fact it additionally exists in right amounts in seaweed, hemp seed, walnuts, kidney beans, soybean and more.

CHAPTER FOUR: FRUITS AND VEGGIES FOR OVERALL PERFORMANCE

While you think of a food plan for building muscle, your mind likely turns to the conventional options. You possibly will cognizance by and large on protein assets like fowl, tuna and eggs. An athlete's weight-reduction plan has to consist of nothing but meta and steamed rice, proper?

However, that is far from the simplest kind of food that's going to be useful for building muscle and improving overall performance. In fact, for bodybuilding, sprinting, swimming, lengthy-distance strolling, and some other sort of athletic pursuit it's far rather important that you get a balanced weight-reduction plan with a view to comprise a wide range of different food corporations. Especially, it is crucial you get your culmination and veggies.

Interested in taking supplements to enhance your athletic performance? What would possibly interest you to learn is that consuming end result and greens can in reality be extra powerful at the same time as also costing plenty less and having a myriad of different exceptional health blessings!

Here are a few examples.

FRUITS AND VEGGIES THAT ENHANCE ATHLETIC OVERALL PERFORMANCE

Beets.

Beets are a long way away from many of the very most important vegetables for building muscle and for athletes of a wide variety.

That's because beets are among the best ingredients in the world in relation to raising nitric oxide. Nitric oxide is a herbal 'vasodilator'. Because of this it could cause the blood vessels (veins and arteries) to dilate (widen) thereby encouraging the glide of oxygen and vitamins across the frame.

The end result is that the muscle groups get greater oxygen and power at some point of education and more vitamins for enhancing recuperation. This may help you carry for more reps, run in additional distances and get better at a faster price.

Potatoes

Carbohydrates are regularly made out to be the bad men but in truth they are very vital for building muscle and for physical training. Potatoes are a very good carbohydrate because they're also excessive in fiber, high in vitamin C (which enhances restoration) and coffee in energy. Consume after a workout and the energy will pass immediately to the muscle groups instead of the waist.

Spinach.

Spinach is a vegetable that is excessive in protein as well as being a great source of phytoecdysteroids. These don't have anything unusual with anabolic steroids however they'll have a comparable effect — with some research suggesting they're a very good option for encouraging muscle constructing and testosterone manufacturing.

Kale

Kale is the vegetable maximum in calcium. Calcium is definitely very important in your exercises, not the simplest does it help to strengthen the bones however it additionally reinforces your connective tissue and it allows to reinforce contractions for greater explosive strength in the course of workouts.

Kale is very modern-day proper now being high in protein and coffee in calories. A shame it feels a bit truthful though!

Mushrooms

Mushrooms are technically no longer culmination or greens, however they are determined in the same aisle and they're safe for vegans, so that they're fair game to include right here. Mushrooms aren't most effective any other high-quality source of protein but also come with a huge variety of extra fitness blessings and blessings. They're packed with minerals, they can inspire recovery from education and lots more besides!

It's actually best a count number of times till we begin seeing mushroom protein shakes cropping up in health stores!

The alternative extremely good benefit of mushrooms is they comprise diet D. In truth, they're one of the few dietary assets of vitamin D! (any other being oily fish).

That is important seeing as nutrition D is considered to be a master hormone regulator, and is chargeable for encouraging the production of testosterone specifically — one of the important anabolic hormones for building muscle and burning fats.

What's extra, is that nutrition D has lately been proven to be plenty more potent than even diet C in relation to assisting the immune system and preventing colds and flush. As any athlete is aware of, a chilly can be sufficient to derail an athlete's training plan, which in flip may be the distinction between victory and failure!

Carrots

Carrots are commonly healthy and a terrific supply of nutrition A, C and okay. What's actually thrilling about them though is the lutein, which can also help to grow energy stages and beautify the efficiency of your mitochondria !

Your mitochondria are the power factories of your cells which convert glucose into ATP (glucose being the sugar that comes from carbs, and ATP being the usable form of strength on your frame). This in a quick way that with carrots and other resources of lutein, you could sincerely run quicker and you'll sincerely burn greater calories even while you're resting !

In one study, rats had been given lutein (which is a source of fats to absorb, consisting of milk) and it became known that they started going for walks long distances voluntarily on their wheel, burning a lot more fats as they did.

Apples

Apples are wealthy in vitamin C, that is every other vital nutrition for reinforcing the immune system and assisting athletes train longer and harder without fail. Vitamin C also facilitates the restore of muscle tissue, will increase serotonin to aid with intellectual recuperation, and even increases the production of both testosterone and nitric oxide whilst paired with zinc.

On pinnacle of all this, apples also are very rich in fiber, which can help to enhance bowel actions, the absorption of food, blood strain, and greater. Fiber is also key to supporting a healthy microbiome, which in flip can support a healthful immune gadget, better temper, weight reduction, and much more.

CHAPTER 5: EXCEPTIONAL SUPERFOOD CULMINATION AND VEGETABLES FOR MOOD, POWER, BEAUTY, AND GREATER

So, you're now not particularly inquisitive about weight reduction? Possibly you're already glad about the scale you are? (proper for you !)

Perhaps you're no longer an athlete? Perhaps you don't have noticeable health problems?

Fruits and vegetables are for absolutely everyone. And just to ram that factor home, here are some greater examples of fruits and vegetables with wildly various exclusive healthful advantages.

BROCCOLI AND LEAFY VEGGIES FOR SPLENDOR AND BEING PREGNANT

Sure, culmination and vegetables can help to make your appearance more beautiful. And that's the actual event of something as easy as your humble broccoli!

Broccoli is perhaps a little less 'exceptional' whilst in comparison with a number of the opposite superfood fruits and veggies on this list. but don't allow that idiot you: this is nevertheless an exceedingly nutritious food that everybody should be getting more of.

For starters, broccoli is a great supply of fiber and may all over again assist to enhance your digestion, your bowel actions, and lots greater. On top of that even though broccoli is likewise very high in vitamin K, vitamin C, fiber, potassium, collagen, iron, calcium, and more.

Allow's start by diving into that collagen. This is something that absolutely everyone wants however very few folks get. Collagen has been shown to enhance mind feature and fight against Alzheimer's, it additionally allows to reduce back ache, improves pores and skin elasticity, strengthens the nails, combats leaky intestine syndrome, fights knee pain, and generally toughens up your tendons, ligaments, and bones.

That is why food, including bone broth, is so noticeably good for us. And now recent studies are suggesting an excellent more effective motive that collagen is probably so important. Researchers now suspect that human beings might once have lived by and large through ingesting bone marrow from animal carcasses. The argument goes that hunter gatherers may also have been sick-equipped to take on massive prey. However, we were excellent at tracking down our prey and following them.

What probably could have happened often, is that we'd have accompanied antelopes and different animals to the factory wherein they were attacked and killed through animals like lions and tigers. They could then have stripped those animals of all their meat, leaving at the back of the skeleton. That's whilst the cunning and ingenious humans could have come along, damaged open the bones with our tactile palms, after which we ate nutritious collagen from inside.

If this is indeed real, then we advanced in an environment wherein we consumed big quantities of the materials of bone. And we now discover ourselves flung into a world in which we very hardly ever get these crucial nutrients. If that's the case, then broccoli may be even greater useful than we at first assumed!

Pregnant moms should simply look into eating greater broccoli and more veggies in standard. That's due to the fact both broccoli and many salad leaves are an awesome source of folate, that is something that everyone moms are endorsed to devour.

Not getting enough folate will increase the risk of headaches in being pregnant, and that's why plenty of mothers will try and get more artificially through using pregnancy dietary supplements.

This is in which it's essential to point out the enormous benefits of having greater vitamins out of your weight loss plan rather than from dietary supplements. Whilst it's authentic that you can benefit from supplements, the clue here is inside the call. Those are intended to supplement your regular food plan.

That is to mention that they should be taken in addition to your everyday weight loss program, in place of as an alternative. Vitamins from your food regimen are far extra powerful than those taken in pill form, as they're combined with several vitamins, fat, fibers, and other elements.

Collectively, those assist to improve absorption of the key factors and that makes them a lot more powerful. The thing to recognize is that the human body developed at the same time as being exposed to those ingredients and consequently is optimally designed to extract the nutritional value on this shape. It isn't always designed to devour vitamins in an artificial form.

This is why so many let you know no longer to take diet drugs on an 'empty stomach'. They simply work better as meals.

CAYENNE PEPPER FOR WEIGHT REDUCTION, TESTOSTERONE, AND EXTRA

Cayenne pepper meanwhile is every other amazing device within the conflict towards infection. This is a compound that makes food highly spiced and is broadly discovered in ointments and lotions because of its anti-irritation results. It's a common ache alleviation too as it depletes nerve cells of the chemical 'substance P'. Substance P reasons each inflammation and the feeling of ache, so that is a super component to feature for your weight-reduction plan in case you do be afflicted by a situation like fibromyalgia or arthritis.

Cayenne additionally comes filled with flavonoids and carotenoids. These are antioxidants that save you cell damage, thereby in addition combating against infection.

Cayenne pepper also has some astounding advantages. It's been proven to be an effective urge for food suppressant, for instance, meaning that if you are someone who struggles to stick to a weight loss plan, you might begin to find it a little less difficult to be disciplined and, thereby, with a bit of luck, see the load start to fall off.

At the same time, cayenne pepper may also assist in enhancing digestion. This is crucial because higher digestion doesn't simply give you extra strength and save you soreness, but it also lets you take in vitamins from your meals. This means that every one of the benefits you're getting from the alternative superfoods on this list will then grow to up to eleven.

What's more, cayenne pepper has additionally been shown to boost testosterone. This route is the hormone that most of us realize is the 'male hormone' and is responsible for the male intercourse power, as well as a number of the variations between ladies and men. Growing testosterone in men will increase muscle tone, reduce fat storage, increase aggression, aid with recuperation, fortify the immune system and more.

Guys who don't get sufficient testosterone will exhibit signs and symptoms of despair, low electricity, low temper, and coffee intercourse power. In addition, they struggle with weight gain and occasional muscle tissue. Conversely, guys with high testosterone exhibit the trends that we accomplish with the conventional 'alpha male' at the side of toned and powerful physiques.

That is why so many guys try to augment their natural testosterone manufacturing through using steroids and different capsules—notwithstanding the ones sporting numerous health warnings and severe risks.

The clearly traumatic component is that testosterone in men is growing throughout the globe by 1% a year. This is partially because of the usage of feminine products and their effect on our water supply, alongside a host of other problems (positive plastics and our generally inactive lifestyles). However, the eating regimen plays a big part in it too. Time to start consuming a touch of much less processed food and a touch of cayenne pepper.

ELDERBERRY FOR INFECTION

Elderberry is a berry that is rich in nutrients. It's once more a fruit that is absent from lots of our everyday diets, and so it's one that you should consider reintroducing.

The simple fact of the problem is that most people rely on an equal number of fruits and vegetables day in and day out. This way, though, we are ensuring we get a lot of nutrients in terms of impact, whilst missing out on a few others. The great food plan is the most varied diet – the only one that includes the most important range of different end results: veggies, meats, herbs, and more. So what can elderberries do for you?

Elderberry has been used since prehistoric instances and has been used as a complement or remedy by a bunch of ancient cultures—together with the historical Egyptians.

Nowadays, we now realize that these fruits are pretty high in flavonoids, especially our pals' anthocyanins—powerful antioxidants like resveratrol.

At the same time, elderberries have been shown to assist in improving the production of cytokines. These are the messenger molecules that our bodies use in order to manipulate the immune system. Pro-inflammatory cytokines assist in encouraging infection at the same time as cytokines help to reduce it. That is all very vital because it essentially ensures that the body is in a position to correctly regulate its personal response to viruses and illnesses and to help heal wounds and accidents.

Many of us suppose that inflammation is always a bad element—in truth, irritation enables us to ruin infections before they have a chance to take impact, as well as to inspire recuperation by way of delivering extra vitamins to the affected area. The hassle is that this response goes haywire.

It turns out that, for similar reasons, elderberries may also be fairly powerful at combating allergic reactions!

At the pinnacle of all this, elderberries are also notably effective at preventing and destroying pathogens, being useful in combating infections, colds, and a number of other troubles. Most thrilling of all, the tiny berries contain amazing antiviral agents that have been proven to simply "deactivate" viruses.

These work by stopping the viruses from being able to interrupt via cellular partitions the usage of their haemagglutinin spikes, which in turn renders them almost inert. They're, for that reason, very effective for combating troubles like rhinitis, as well as stopping them from occurring in the first place. Of course, there's additionally the standard diet and mineral content, which you generally tend to get from berries.

CHAPTER 6: HOW ANTIOXIDANTS ASSIST YOU TO LIVE LONGER

Antioxidants are determined obviously in our food regimen and also are a key characteristic of many supplements. Antioxidants are something of a buzz phrase in recent times and antioxidant vitamins and minerals as well as a variety of Naka Herb dietary supplements are tremendously popular.

What is the motive for this? And what exactly are antioxidants? Here we will look a little at how a mobile works, how a mobile dies, and why antioxidants are so important.

Our cells are made from various parts, but all you want to realize approximately in this instance is the mobile wall and the nucleus. The cellular wall, surrounded by mitochondria, is the part of the mobile that holds the whole thing together and gives the cell its spherical look.

Meanwhile, the nucleus is the middle of the cell, which is frequently known as the "control middle". Right here is wherein the DNA is stored, the 'blueprint' that tells the cell what it looks like, how to behave and where the alternative essential cells move in the body.

Sadly, though, what's additionally in our body is "unfastened radicals", and this is where the antioxidant vitamins and minerals and the Naka Herb dietary supplements come in. Basically, unfastened radicals are substances that travel across the body and harm the cells. There are many things, from truly respiratory (oxygen is reactive and damages cells) to getting an excessive amount of direct sunlight (the UV waves in sunlight are radioactive and can damage our mobile walls too).

These free radicals then do a lot of critical harm within the frame and are sufficient to eventually make our skin appear older - because the harm, even if microscopic, can eventually add up to be seen with the naked eye, and this also applies to pores and skin cells.That is why lots of exposure to the sun will make you look tanned and precise in a short time, but in the long run, it will result in your pores and skin acting wrinkled and leathery.

However, ultimately, these free radicals will damage all the way through the mobile partitions, and this could mean that they will attain the nucleus where the DNA is housed. In the event that they reach this, then they are able to cause damage to your actual genetic code and this results in mutation which alters the expression of the mobile and renders it unable to do its job.

Because cells reproduce by means of splitting (mitosis), this method means that after the cellular splits, it's going to reproduce the DNA across and you will have two fault cells. Your immune system tries to prevent this and may be aided if you buy herbs online, but it would be preferable if it could be avoided.Due to the fact that those useless cells as they unfold end up cancerous and can ultimately cause the failure of whole organs.

Antioxidant nutrients and minerals from fruits, vegetables, or even dietary supplements will help you to do that by way of destroying the free radicals on effect, thereby preventing them from ever causing that damage. These will then slow your visible aging and help to prevent most cancers—no longer bad!

CHAPTER 7: A WAY TO USE FRUITS AND VEGGIES TO EFFICIENTLY IMPROVE YOUR FITNESS

At this point, you need to have a comprehensive idea of the quality factors to make certain you are getting enough end result and greens in your eating regimen. Those can enhance your health in a myriad of ways, and if you are presently feeling worn-out, moody, ill, or even depressed, it's exceedingly likely that you have a deficiency in at least one of these micronutrients. And this must come as no wonder—for the reason that the giant majority of humans do have some kind of deficiency these days.

The next query is the way you ought to be lightly integrating these fruits and greens. Are there any drawbacks? How many do you want precisely? Are you able to just use a diet tablet alternatively?

What number of end results and veggies do you actually need?

You might have heard that you should aim to eat at least five one-of-a-kind combinations and vegetables a day. This is a piece of well-known advice that is given by many fitness organizations and governments. Some agencies have improved this range to seven. It is the right advice, but it's also arbitrary.

What do I imply by way of that? Essentially, that means it's based on nothing!

Fruits and veggies are not inherently good for you. They're not right for you because they are fruits and veggies. As a substitute, they're best for you because they include all the essential micronutrients.

The micronutrients are required in one-of-a-kind quantities and types, and ultimately, the most important thing we can do for our fitness is just to get as many of them as possible. The more fruits and veggies you devour, the higher you get. And it is very difficult to overdose while you get your nutrients from herbal sources like this.

And be very dubious when a packet of meals tells you it counts as "certainly one of your five a day." If that food is enormously processed, then probabilities are it won't have many vitamins in it at all anymore. At the very least, it's likely to be a whole lot lower in fiber. Hence, the advantages won't be as excellent as they could have been had you eaten up that nutrient itself. Use common sense, and eat as many complete, real-end results and vegetables as possible!

THE DANGERS OF TOO MANY FRUITS AND VEGETABLES

That said, you can do yourself harm by eating too many fruits and vegetables. Or to be a touch extra unique, it's far more notably clean to cause damage via eating an excessive amount of fruit. That's because fruit is noticeably acidic and full of sugar. Both these things make it negative for your enamel specifically. Many folks that switch to diets that are mainly focused on the usage of smoothies will turn out to have extreme tooth problems!

One approach to this is to avoid consuming an excessive amount of fruit juice or too many fruit smoothies. Alternatively, cognizance on ingesting vegetable smoothies, which usually contain plenty of sugar.

Another consideration is that end results and greens are still a source of energy. This is especially authentic for things like avocados, which have become all the rage lately. Avocados are first rate for enhancing testosterone (thanks to their healthy saturated fat content), and at the same time as they may be beneficial for those looking to avoid carbs, they could still make you fat!

Don't make the mistake of thinking that "fruits and veggies are healthy and, consequently, can't make you fat."

The truth is that they nevertheless include energy, and you still need to listen to music and manage your energy to keep away from unwanted weight gain.

CHAPTER 8: GROWING A WEIGHT LOSS PLAN RICH IN FRUITS AND VEGGIES

So, you need to be eating greater fruits and greens, and we've seen already that there are a huge range of precise meals which have a specially remarkable gain – just as there are a huge range of particular nutrients and minerals which you want to try to search for in your weight loss plan.

However, how do you go about enforcing that plan? How do you go from suffering to getting your 5 a day to being able to consume a vast array of various beneficial components without difficulty?

Due to the fact that's the other key element to realize: you shouldn't be taking a reductive technique of seeking to look for each item individually. If you try this, then you'll find that you grow to be spending a huge amount of money, and in the end now not getting lots gain.

This book has indexed a massive quantity of end results and greens that you could be trying to find out especially on the way to enjoy advantages on your beauty, in your energy ranges, for infection, for immunity...you may therefore be tempted to assume you may choose and pick out the blessings you want! But that is the wrong technique.

When there are that many distinct superfoods that each offer some type of exceptional advantage, you truly can not searching for out every one in my view. That is in particular proper seeing as a lot of them won't blend collectively, many aren't to be had on your local supermarket, and a few will handiest be fit for human consumption for a short quantity of time. So, what do you do as an alternative?

THE STRATEGY: THE PURPOSE IS VARIETY

As opposed to seeking out individual exceptional fruits and vegetables, what is some distance most advantageous is to truly aim to get the largest variety you likely can to your diet. With the aid of doing this, you will cowl the biggest spectrum of elements, and thereby get the most important variety of various benefits from your eating regimen.

You may find the healthiest superfood vegetable inside the international market, but if that becomes all you ate you then wouldn't get all that lots of advantage – because you'd most effectively be getting big quantities of these same elements.

We don't consider meals such as apples as being superfoods, but because they contain massive amounts of vitamin C (antioxidants, boosts testosterone, encourages nitric oxide formation, produces serotonin), and epicatechin, they may be just as brilliant as those greater wonderful ideas.

Furthermore, in case you eat 3 specific fruits and vegetables, then the range of nutrients you get might be way more.
Research shows as well, that our microbiome – the healthy bacteria residing in our guts – gain most of all from a various weight loss plan. The greater the variety of ingredients you consume, the stronger your intestine fitness might be – resulting in weight reduction, more energy, better temper, and more.

Eventually, with the aid of aiming to simply "devour masses of end result and veggies" you can lessen the quantity of ideas this eating regimen raises, which in flip will help you to be much more likely to paste to your new dedication.

HOW TO INCREASE FRUIT AND VEGETABLE VARIETY

So how do you increase the variety? Here are some simple ideas to help you accomplish this without adding too many strains to your next shopping trip:

- Make lots of stews, warm pots, and Italian dishes. in case you're cooking something like a bolognaise, then it's surely very clean to just throw a group of end result and veggies right into a pot with some mince.

- To make this even easier, attempt grating such things as carrots (so that you don't want to peel them), and use frozen elements like mushrooms, peas, and sweetcorn.

- Make lots of salads! An easy way to make a chilly lunch is to get a few salad leaves, throw on some sweet potatoes, slice a few cucumbers, and add a pinch of lemon. This could be served at the side of almost anything you prepare for dinner. Pick out small-leaf spinach and you'll get iron and folate. Then just vary which leaf you use each time.

- Freeze! While doing this, cook up massive batches of meals and then freeze them in plenty of, in my view, portioned tupperwares. Then all you want to do is to defrost each one as you come to consume it.

- Make smoothies! These are extraordinarily easy to provide – simply throw a group of fruits and/or vegetables in and hit the combo. They also offer a big range of super benefits. Some of the most lively and cheerful people I know devour daily smoothies.

- I purchase fruits and vegetables. Lots of cafes promote fruits at the counter, and the same is true in many grocers. Instead of purchasing a chocolatey snack, simply purchase the most extraordinary-looking fruit you can find!

CHAPTER NINE: WHAT ABOUT MULTIVITAMIN SUPPLEMENTS ?

If the primary benefits of fruits and vegetables come from the vitamins, minerals, and different vital micronutrients, then you definitely might have a completely reasonable query: what about multivitamins?

A multivitamin complement is a supplement that includes a balance of various nutrients. You might typically see one that carries an aggregate of diet C, D, A, and B complex. Likewise, multimineral supplements would possibly contain Iron, Magnesium, Potassium, Calcium, and Zinc for "healthful bones and hormone stability."

Are these merchandise just as desirable as the "actual deal?"

Yes and no.

On the one hand, you could soak up an advantage from dietary supplements. Some people will tell you that this isn't actual, however there are numerous top motives to believe otherwise. For one, did you recognize that there simply exist numerous merchandise which can be designed to update your entire weight loss program? These include the likes of Soylent, which supposedly contains every single nutrient the frame desires, all balanced flawlessly.

Is it a very good idea? By no means! But the thing to notice right now's that individuals who use this product live to tell the tale...

and they're certainly quite wholesome! And with that in mind, we can therefore claim that multivitamins also can be absorbed.

But there's a catch. The primary of these catches is that a multivitamin is best going to be as correct as the individual that designed it. We noticed with lutein and different fat soluble vitamins for example. These want a source of fat so one can be absorbed into the bloodstream. Get them from herbal meals sources, and chances are that the source of fats may be covered. Get them from a vitamin complement and that they might not.

Similar interactions additionally exist among many different vitamins and minerals, where one will help the opposite to be absorbed more effortlessly. Likewise, one of a kind vitamins and minerals soak up at one-of-a-kind prices, and so ideally shouldn't be blended right into a single product.

Then there are all the different matters that fruits and veggies comprise that do us top – consisting of fiber, amino acids, and more. PLUS there's the small truth that all fruits and veggies comprise materials that we don't absolutely understand or possibly aren't even aware about.

We most effectively just located the awesome benefits of lutein (that move past eye health). So consuming actual fruit and greens is usually optimum.

However with that stated, if the choice comes right down to the usage of a supplement or not getting those useful vitamins at all… then the supplement is of path higher. In truth, a Supplement may be a very convenient and easy manner to get what you need for your weight loss plan, or can be considered as a "return up."

CHAPTER 10: YOUR BLUEPRINT FOR GREATER HEALTH

And with that, we attain the quit of this manual. At this factor, you have to now have a much higher concept of precisely which culmination and greens you need on your weight-reduction plan, which of them can provide the most advantages, and the way it's surely the style of this stuff that trumps everything else.

Likewise, you should now have an understanding of the first-rate methods to get those fruits and veggies on your eating regimen, and the satisfactory methods to keep away from any troubles that can come from them.

With all that stated, right here is your blueprint to enhance your fitness and happiness vastly with the aid of getting more fruits and vegetables:

- begin your day with a smoothie, but don't have more than one fruit smoothie
- Don't aim to get simply 5-7 fruits and greens to your weight loss plan. Get as many as you may which will get a numerous mix.
- Use a complement as a "returned up." This is additionally particularly beneficial while looking for more difficult to understand and rare nutrients.
- however ensure that you read the instructions and do your very own studies. you could want to think about timing and

adding a supply of fat to aid absorption.

- Use techniques to make it as smooth as feasible to get greater fruits and greens to your weight loss plan · keep away from processed foods and "empty energy" – replace such things as chips and chocolate bars with salads and carrotsticks
- keep this software for 30 days. You must discover you note you have greater strength, drive, and higher health.
- Use this new power to enhance your way of life in other methods!

BOOKS BY THIS AUTHOR

Colouring Art Collection Anti-Stress For Children: Colouring Art Collection Anti-Stress

Experience a fun and whimsical fantasy adventure with this delightful children coloring book!
Would you want to unwind and appreciate line art designs? Looking for a fresh, original coloring book to inspire your imagination and give you the chance to practice mindfulness? Then you should read this book!
This book has something for everyone thanks to the fantastical mushrooms and toadstools, vibrant and exciting scenes, and loads of animals as well.
Coloring book information

70 hand-drawn illustrations specifically created to inspire your creative aspirations
Printed on separate sheets to avoid bleed-through and make it simple for you to remove and frame your favorites!
suitable for watercolors, colored pencils, fine-liners, gel pens, markers, and gel pens
Every skill level is catered for with a variety of easy and complicated drawings, and there are endless hours of coloring fun and mental relaxation.
So this book is for you if you're seeking for a silly and enjoyable fantasy journey to help you get lost in the world of coloring!

www.ingramcontent.com/pod-product-compliance
Lightning Source LLC
Chambersburg PA
CBHW072130150726

47999CB00005B/2217